LED Light Therapy Guide for Beginners

Benefits of LED Light Therapy

By

Clyde Artair

Table of Contents

CHAPTER 1

Introduction

1.1 What is LED Light Therapy

LED (Light Emitting Diode) Light Therapy, often referred to as photobiomodulation or low-level light therapy, is a non-invasive and painless medical treatment that utilizes specific wavelengths of light to stimulate the skin, tissues, and cells for therapeutic purposes. It has gained popularity in recent years as a versatile and effective approach to addressing a wide range of skin and health concerns.

LED Light Therapy involves the use of LED devices that emit different colors of light, each with its unique properties and benefits. These devices can be used in various settings, from professional clinical treatments to at-home devices, making it accessible to a broad audience. LED Light Therapy is often used in the fields of dermatology, aesthetics, and general wellness.

The core concept behind LED Light Therapy is that different colors of light can penetrate the skin at various depths and interact with cells, promoting various biological responses. Each color of light is absorbed by different components in the skin, which can result in numerous therapeutic effects. This non-invasive nature of the treatment makes it suitable for people of all ages and skin types, and it has minimal risks or side effects when used as directed.

1.2 Benefits of LED Light Therapy

LED Light Therapy offers a wide array of potential benefits, making it a versatile option for those seeking improved skin health and well-being. Some of the primary benefits include:

1. **Skin Rejuvenation:** LED Light Therapy can help stimulate collagen production, reduce fine lines and wrinkles, and improve skin texture, giving the skin a more youthful and radiant appearance.

2. **Acne Management:** The blue and red-light wavelengths can target and kill the bacteria responsible for acne breakouts while reducing inflammation and promoting healing.

3. **Pain Relief:** LED Light Therapy is used in pain management to reduce inflammation, alleviate muscle and joint pain, and support tissue recovery, making it valuable for athletes and those with chronic pain conditions.

4. **Wound Healing:** It can accelerate the body's natural wound healing processes, which is particularly beneficial for post-surgical recovery and wound care.

5. **Hair Growth:** Certain wavelengths of LED light have shown promise in promoting hair growth and combatting hair loss in both men and women.

6. **Psoriasis and Eczema Relief:**
LED Therapy can help manage
the symptoms of skin
conditions like psoriasis and
eczema by reducing
inflammation and promoting
healthier skin.

7. **Mood and Sleep
Improvement:** Some people
have reported improvements in
mood and sleep patterns with
the use of specific LED light
colors, particularly in the form
of light therapy lamps or
devices designed for this
purpose.

8. **Overall Skin Health:** LED
Light Therapy can enhance skin
clarity, reduce redness and
pigmentation, and help balance
skin tone.

1.3 How Does LED Light Therapy Work

The mechanism of action behind LED Light Therapy is rooted in the interaction between different wavelengths of light and the cells and tissues of the body. Here's a simplified breakdown of how it works:

- **Absorption of Light:** Different colors of light penetrate the skin at varying depths. Red light, for example, can penetrate more deeply than blue light. When the light reaches the skin, it is absorbed by specific molecules or chromophores within the cells.

- **Stimulation of Mitochondria:** The absorbed light energy stimulates the mitochondria, the powerhouse of the cell, to produce more adenosine triphosphate (ATP), which is the primary energy source for cellular activities. This boost in ATP production enhances cellular function and can lead to a range of therapeutic effects.

- **Cellular Responses:** Depending on the color of light used, different cellular responses are triggered. For instance, red light is associated with increased collagen production and improved blood circulation, while blue light is known for its antibacterial properties and its ability to target and destroy acne-causing bacteria.

- **Reduction of Inflammation:** LED Light Therapy can reduce inflammation, which is a common factor in many skin conditions and pain-related issues. By minimizing inflammation, it can help alleviate symptoms and promote healing.

- **Healing and Regeneration:** The enhanced cellular function, reduced inflammation, and stimulation of various processes contribute to wound healing, tissue repair, and overall skin rejuvenation.

It's important to note that while LED Light Therapy offers numerous benefits, results may vary from person to person, and consistency in treatment is often required to achieve the desired outcomes. Additionally, safety precautions and choosing the appropriate wavelengths for specific concerns are crucial to maximize the therapeutic effects while minimizing any potential risks.

CHAPTER 2

Understanding Different Types of LED Lights

2.1 Red Light Therapy

Red Light Therapy, also known as Low-Level Laser Therapy (LLLT) or Photobiomodulation, utilizes red or near-infrared light with wavelengths typically ranging from 630 to 850 nanometers. This type of therapy has gained immense popularity due to its wide range of applications and therapeutic benefits. Here's an overview of Red Light Therapy:

- **Collagen Production:** Red light penetrates the skin's surface and stimulates the production of collagen, a crucial protein for maintaining skin's elasticity and youthfulness. This leads to reduced wrinkles and improved skin texture.

- **Wound Healing:** Red light promotes cellular regeneration and can accelerate the healing of wounds, cuts, and surgical incisions. It does so by enhancing blood circulation and minimizing inflammation at the cellular level.

- **Pain Relief:** It can be used to alleviate muscle and joint pain. This is achieved by reducing inflammation and promoting the release of endorphins, the body's natural painkillers.

- **Anti-Inflammatory:** Red light has anti-inflammatory properties, making it useful for conditions where inflammation plays a role, such as arthritis.

- **Hair Growth:** In the field of aesthetics, Red Light Therapy has shown promise in stimulating hair growth and reducing hair loss.

2.2 Blue Light Therapy

Blue Light Therapy employs blue light wavelengths typically in the range of 405 to 470 nanometers. It is primarily known for its effectiveness in treating skin conditions, particularly acne. Here are the key points regarding Blue Light Therapy:

- **Acne Treatment:** Blue light is used to target the Propionibacterium acnes bacteria, which plays a significant role in the development of acne. When exposed to blue light, the bacteria's ability to proliferate and cause inflammation is reduced, leading to a decrease in acne lesions.

- **Non-Invasive:** Blue Light Therapy is a non-invasive alternative to topical and oral acne treatments. It is especially valuable for individuals who may be sensitive to or cannot tolerate certain medications.

- **Minimal Side Effects:** When used as directed, Blue Light Therapy has minimal side effects, making it a safer option for acne treatment compared to some pharmaceuticals.

2.3 Green Light Therapy

Green Light Therapy employs wavelengths ranging from approximately 515 to 525 nanometers. While it may not be as commonly recognized as red or blue light therapy, it offers its unique set of benefits:

- **Skin Tone Correction:** Green Light Therapy is often used to address issues related to skin pigmentation, such as hyperpigmentation and melasma. It can help reduce the appearance of brown spots and uneven skin tone.

- **Calming Effect:** Green light has a calming and soothing effect on the skin. It can help reduce redness and inflammation, making it suitable for individuals with sensitive or easily irritated skin.

- **Combination Therapy:** Green light is sometimes used in combination with other colors, such as red or blue, to address multiple skin concerns simultaneously. For instance, it can be used to reduce post-inflammatory redness following Blue Light Therapy for acne.

It's important to note that the effectiveness of LED Light Therapy, regardless of the color of light used, depends on factors such as the specific condition being treated, the choice of the correct wavelength, treatment duration, and consistency. Consulting with a healthcare professional or dermatologist is advisable for a personalized treatment plan, especially for more complex skin issues.

2.4 Yellow Light Therapy

Yellow Light Therapy is a less common but still valuable form of LED Light Therapy that utilizes wavelengths typically in the range of 570 to 590 nanometers. It offers several potential benefits:

- **Reduction of Redness:** Yellow light can help reduce the appearance of redness in the skin, making it suitable for individuals with conditions like rosacea or general skin redness.

- **Improved Lymphatic Function:** It is believed to promote lymphatic flow, which can assist in detoxifying the skin and reducing puffiness.

- **Enhanced Cellular Exchange:** Yellow light therapy is thought to facilitate the exchange of nutrients and waste products between skin cells, potentially leading to healthier and more radiant skin.

- **Combination with Other Colors:** Yellow light can be used in combination with other LED light colors for more comprehensive therapy, often alongside red or green light to address a range of skin concerns.

2.5 Combination LED Therapy

Combination LED Therapy, as the name suggests, involves the use of multiple colors of LED light in a single treatment session. This approach can provide a broader range of benefits and target various skin issues simultaneously. Here are some key aspects of Combination LED Therapy:

- **Customized Treatments:** Combination therapy allows for the customization of treatments to address the unique needs and concerns of an individual's skin. For example, a session might involve red light for collagen production, blue light for acne management, and green light for reducing redness.

- **Synergistic Effects:** The synergy between different wavelengths can enhance the therapeutic outcomes. For instance, combining red and blue light can not only reduce acne but also improve overall skin texture and appearance.

- **Efficient Time Management:** Instead of separate sessions for each type of LED light, combination therapy can save time and offer convenience to those with busy schedules.

- **Professional Guidance:** Combination therapy often requires professional guidance, as the correct selection of wavelengths and their respective treatment durations is crucial for safety and effectiveness.

- **At-Home Devices:** Some at-home LED therapy devices are designed for combination therapy, allowing users to switch between different light colors for a versatile approach to skincare.

It's important to remember that the effectiveness of Combination LED Therapy, as with individual colors of LED light, depends on several factors, including the specific skin issues being addressed and the expertise of the practitioner or user. Always follow professional advice or device instructions when considering combination therapy to ensure the best results while minimizing any potential risks.

CHAPTER 3

Choosing the Right LED Light Therapy Device

3.1 Home Devices vs. Professional Treatments

LED Light Therapy is available in both professional clinical settings and as at-home devices. The choice between the two depends on individual preferences, needs, and resources. Here's a comparison of home devices and professional treatments:

Home Devices:

- **Convenience:** Home devices offer the convenience of using LED therapy at your own schedule and in the comfort of your home. This can be particularly appealing for those with busy lifestyles.

- **Cost-Effective:** Over time, home devices can be more cost-effective compared to multiple professional sessions, especially if you are consistent with your treatments.

- **Privacy:** You can maintain your privacy and treat your skin concerns without the need for regular visits to a clinic or spa.

Professional Treatments:

- **Expert Guidance:** Professional treatments are administered by trained practitioners who can tailor the treatment to your specific needs and provide expert guidance.

- **More Intensive:** Professional treatments often use higher-intensity devices, which can lead to quicker results for certain conditions.

- **Safety and Supervision:** Professional settings ensure that the treatment is administered safely and effectively, reducing the risk of errors or misuse.

- **Combination Therapies:** Clinics and spas often offer combination therapies,

combining LED Light Therapy
with other treatments like
microneedling or chemical
peels for enhanced results.

The choice between home devices and
professional treatments depends on
your goals, budget, and the severity of
your skin concerns. Some individuals
opt for a combination of both, using
home devices for maintenance
between professional sessions.

3.2 Factors to Consider When Buying an LED Device

When considering the purchase of an
LED Light Therapy device for home
use, there are several important
factors to keep in mind:

- **Wavelengths:** Ensure the device emits the appropriate wavelengths of light for your specific skin concern. Different colors of light have different therapeutic effects, so choose a device that aligns with your needs.

- **Intensity and Power:** Consider the power and intensity of the device. Devices with higher power may be more effective for some conditions but should be used with caution and following guidelines to prevent adverse effects.

- **Treatment Area:** Check the treatment area that the device covers. Some devices are designed for specific facial areas, while others can be used on the entire body.

- **Safety Features:** Look for safety features such as timers, eye protection, and temperature control to prevent overexposure or injury.

- **Ease of Use:** Consider how user-friendly the device is, especially if you are new to LED Light Therapy. Clear instructions and ease of operation are important.

- **Quality and Brand Reputation:** Research the brand and read reviews to ensure you are investing in a quality device. Reputable brands are more likely to produce effective and safe products.

- **Price and Warranty:** Compare prices and check for

warranties or return policies.
While quality is important, it's
also important to stay within
your budget.

3.3 Safety Precautions and Certifications

Before purchasing or using any LED
Light Therapy device, it's crucial to
consider safety precautions and
certifications:

- **Eye Protection:** Always wear
  the provided eye protection or
  keep your eyes closed when
  using the device. Direct
  exposure to LED light can be
  harmful to the eyes.

- **Consultation:** If you have
  underlying medical conditions
  or are using the device for a
  specific medical concern,

consult with a healthcare professional or dermatologist for guidance.

- **Certifications:** Check if the device has been certified by relevant authorities to ensure it meets safety and efficacy standards.

- **Skin Sensitivity:** Be aware of your skin's sensitivity. Some individuals may experience irritation or adverse effects, so it's important to start with shorter sessions and lower intensity.

- **Maintenance:** Follow the manufacturer's maintenance instructions to keep the device in good working condition.

- **Pregnancy and Medications:** If you are pregnant or taking certain medications, consult with a healthcare provider to determine whether LED Light Therapy is safe for you.

By carefully considering these factors and adhering to safety precautions, you can choose the right LED Light Therapy device for your needs and use it safely and effectively.

CHAPTER 4

Preparing for Your LED Light Therapy Session

4.1 Skin Preparation

Proper skin preparation is essential to maximize the effectiveness of your LED Light Therapy session and minimize the risk of adverse reactions. Here's what you need to do before your session:

- **Cleanse Your Skin:** Start with clean, makeup-free skin. Use a gentle, non-alcoholic cleanser to remove any dirt, makeup, or skincare products from your face. This ensures that the LED light can penetrate your skin effectively.

- **Exfoliation (Optional):** Depending on your skin type and condition, you may choose to exfoliate before your session. Exfoliation can remove dead skin cells, allowing the LED light to reach deeper layers of the skin. However, be gentle, and avoid aggressive exfoliation, which may irritate the skin.

- **Dry Your Skin:** Ensure that your skin is completely dry before starting the LED Light Therapy session. Moisture on the skin's surface can interfere with the penetration of light.

- **Eye Protection:** If your LED device requires eye protection, put it on before starting the session. Direct exposure to the LED light can be harmful to your eyes.

- **Remove Metal and Jewelry:** Take off any metal objects or jewelry that might reflect or interfere with the light.

4.2 Setting Up the Session Environment

Creating the right environment for your LED Light Therapy session contributes to a more comfortable and effective experience. Here's how to set up your session environment:

- **Quiet and Comfortable Space:** Find a quiet and

comfortable area where you can relax during the session. It's a great opportunity for self-care, so create a calming atmosphere.

- **Privacy:** Ensure you have privacy, especially if you're using an at-home device. You may want to close curtains or doors to create a personal sanctuary.

- **Avoid Distractions:** Minimize distractions such as phone calls, loud noises, or interruptions during the session. This will allow you to fully unwind.

- **Positioning:** Sit or lie down comfortably, and make sure you have easy access to your LED device. You'll need to be in close proximity to it during the session.

- **LED Device Placement:** Position the LED device at the recommended distance from your skin. This information is typically provided in the device's user manual. Follow these guidelines to ensure the appropriate intensity of light.

4.3 Duration and Frequency

The duration and frequency of your LED Light Therapy sessions can vary based on your goals and the specific device you're using. Here are some general guidelines:

- **Duration:** LED Light Therapy sessions typically last between 10 to 30 minutes, although some may be shorter or longer, depending on the device and treatment purpose. Follow the manufacturer's recommendations for the recommended session duration.

- **Frequency:** The frequency of your sessions depends on the issue you're addressing. For general skin health and maintenance, 2-3 sessions per week may be sufficient. For specific skin concerns, such as acne or wrinkle reduction, daily or more frequent sessions may be recommended initially, with less frequent maintenance sessions later.

- **Patience:** Results may take time. Be patient and consistent with your sessions. It can take several weeks or even months to see significant improvements, especially for skin conditions like acne or fine lines.

- **Consultation:** If you're unsure about the optimal duration and frequency for your specific needs, consult with a dermatologist or a skincare professional. They can provide personalized guidance.

LED Light Therapy is generally safe when used as directed, but it's important to follow the recommendations of the manufacturer and consult a healthcare professional if you have any concerns or specific skin issues to address.

CHAPTER 5

How to Perform LED Light Therapy

5.1 Step-by-Step Instructions

Performing LED Light Therapy at home or in a professional setting involves several key steps to ensure a safe and effective session. Here are step-by-step instructions:

Step 1: Skin Preparation

- Ensure your skin is clean and free from makeup, dirt, and skincare products. Cleanse your face using a gentle, non-

alcoholic cleanser. If
exfoliation is part of your
skincare routine, perform it
before cleansing.

Step 2: Eye Protection

- If your LED device requires
  eye protection, put it on to
  shield your eyes from direct
  exposure to the light.

Step 3: Positioning

- Sit or lie down comfortably in a
  quiet and private space where
  you won't be disturbed during
  the session.

Step 4: Turn on the LED Device

- Turn on your LED device
  following the manufacturer's
  instructions. Some devices may
  allow you to select the specific
  light color or treatment mode.

Step 5: Appropriate Distance

- Position the LED device at the recommended distance from your skin. This distance is typically provided in the device's user manual. Follow these guidelines to ensure the optimal intensity of light for your skin.

Step 6: Start the Session

- Start the LED Light Therapy session by activating the device. Ensure that the light is evenly distributed over the targeted area. Hold the device steady throughout the session.

Step 7: Relax and Enjoy

- Relax and enjoy the session. You can use this time to

meditate, listen to soothing
music, or simply unwind.

Step 8: Session Duration

- Stick to the recommended
  session duration, typically
  ranging from 10 to 30 minutes,
  depending on the device and
  treatment purpose.

Step 9: Turn Off the Device

- Once the session is complete,
  turn off the LED device.
  Follow the manufacturer's
  instructions for proper
  shutdown.

Step 10: Skin Care

- After your session, you can
  apply your usual skincare
  products, such as moisturizers
  or serums, if desired. The LED

treatment often enhances the absorption of these products.

5.2 Targeted Areas and Techniques

The effectiveness of LED Light Therapy can vary depending on the targeted areas and specific techniques used:

Facial Skin:

- For general skin rejuvenation, focus the LED device on your entire face. Move the device in slow, circular motions to ensure even coverage.

Acne-Prone Areas:

- If targeting acne, direct the LED light toward the affected areas, especially those prone to breakouts. Hold the device still

for a few seconds on each acne
spot.

Wrinkles and Fine Lines:

- To address wrinkles and fine
  lines, concentrate the LED light
  on areas where signs of aging
  are prominent, such as around
  the eyes (crow's feet), mouth,
  and forehead. Gently glide the
  device over these areas.

Hair Growth:

- If using LED therapy for hair
  growth, move the device slowly
  over the scalp, making sure the
  light reaches the hair follicles.
  Part your hair to access the
  scalp.

Pain Relief and Muscles:

- For pain relief and muscle
  recovery, direct the LED light

to the affected area. Keep the device at a consistent distance and adjust the intensity as needed.

Full Body Treatment:

- Some LED devices are designed for full-body treatment. Follow the manufacturer's instructions for recommended techniques to cover larger areas like the back or legs.

Consistency is key: Regardless of the targeted areas, consistency in your LED Light Therapy sessions is essential for achieving the desired results. Follow the recommended frequency and duration for your specific concerns and adjust your technique as needed.

Always follow the manufacturer's guidelines and consult with a healthcare professional or dermatologist if you have specific skin conditions or concerns. Additionally, adhere to safety precautions and use the device as directed to minimize risks and maximize benefits.

CHAPTER 6
Skin Conditions and LED Light Therapy

6.1 Acne and Acne Scars

Acne:

LED Light Therapy is a promising option for individuals dealing with acne. Here's how it can help:

- **Bacteria Reduction:** Blue light (typically in the 405-470 nanometer range) targets and destroys the Propionibacterium acnes bacteria responsible for acne breakouts. By reducing the presence of this bacteria, LED light therapy can lead to a decrease in acne lesions.

- **Inflammation Reduction:** LED therapy, especially blue and red light, can minimize the inflammation associated with acne, making it effective for both active breakouts and preventing future ones.

- **Faster Healing:** The enhanced cellular function and increased blood flow promoted by LED light therapy can speed up the body's natural healing processes, helping acne lesions heal more quickly.

Acne Scars:

While LED Light Therapy may not directly remove acne scars, it can improve the overall quality of your skin, which can help make scars less noticeable. Here's how it can assist with acne scars:

- **Collagen Stimulation:** Red light therapy (wavelengths around 630-850 nanometers) can stimulate collagen production, which can plump up the skin, making scars appear less deep and noticeable over time.

- **Improved Skin Texture:** By promoting healthier skin, LED therapy can help improve the overall texture of your skin, potentially making scars appear less prominent.

- **Preventing New Acne:** Continued LED therapy can help manage acne and prevent new breakouts, which can minimize the formation of additional acne scars.

It's important to note that LED Light Therapy is most effective for milder to moderate cases of acne. For severe acne, consult with a dermatologist who may recommend a combination of treatments, including LED therapy.

6.2 Wrinkles and Fine Lines

Wrinkles and fine lines are common signs of skin aging. LED Light Therapy can be a valuable tool in addressing these concerns:

- **Collagen Production:** Red light therapy, in particular, is known for stimulating collagen production. Collagen is essential for maintaining skin elasticity, and increased collagen can help reduce the appearance of wrinkles and fine lines.

- **Improved Skin Texture:** LED therapy can enhance skin texture, making it smoother and more youthful in appearance.

- **Reduction in Inflammation:** By minimizing inflammation, LED therapy can also help reduce puffiness and redness associated with aging skin.

- **Maintenance:** LED therapy can be used as part of a regular skincare routine to maintain the results of other anti-aging treatments like chemical peels or microdermabrasion.

- **Prevention:** LED therapy can be a proactive approach to prevent the formation of wrinkles and fine lines, especially when used regularly.

While LED Light Therapy can be effective for addressing fine lines and wrinkles, it's essential to be consistent with treatments and understand that results may take time. Additionally, a comprehensive skincare routine that includes sun protection, proper hydration, and quality skincare products can complement LED therapy for optimal anti-aging benefits.

6.3 Hyperpigmentation

Hyperpigmentation refers to the darkening of certain areas of the skin, often due to excess melanin production. LED Light Therapy can be a helpful tool in managing hyperpigmentation. Here's how it can be beneficial:

- **Reduced Pigment Production:** Some types of LED light, especially green light, can help reduce melanin production, which is responsible for hyperpigmentation. This can lead to a more even skin tone.

- **Increased Cellular Activity:** LED therapy promotes increased cellular activity and turnover, which can help shed pigmented skin cells and replace them with healthier, evenly pigmented ones.

- **Combination with Topical Products:** LED therapy can

enhance the effectiveness of topical skincare products designed for hyperpigmentation, as it increases the absorption of these products into the skin.

To effectively address hyperpigmentation, it's essential to be consistent with LED Light Therapy sessions and combine it with sun protection, a suitable skincare routine, and possibly the guidance of a dermatologist for more severe cases.

6.4 Rosacea

Rosacea is a chronic skin condition characterized by redness, flushing, and visible blood vessels. While LED Light Therapy may not cure rosacea, it can help manage some of its symptoms:

- **Redness Reduction:** Green and yellow light can be used to reduce redness associated with rosacea. These wavelengths have anti-inflammatory properties and can soothe the skin.

- **Calming Effect:** LED therapy can have a calming effect on rosacea-prone skin, reducing irritation and discomfort.

- **Combination with Topical Products:** LED therapy can complement the use of topical products prescribed by a dermatologist for rosacea management.

It's crucial to consult with a dermatologist for a comprehensive rosacea treatment plan. LED therapy can be a part of that plan, but the condition often requires a multifaceted approach for optimal results.

6.5 Wound Healing

LED Light Therapy has shown considerable promise in promoting wound healing. Here's how it can be valuable in this context:

- **Stimulated Cellular Regeneration:** LED therapy, particularly red and near-infrared light, stimulates cellular regeneration, which is crucial for wound healing.

- **Enhanced Blood Circulation:** Increased blood circulation, facilitated by LED therapy, delivers oxygen and nutrients to the wound area, expediting the healing process.

- **Reduced Inflammation:** LED therapy can reduce inflammation in the wound area, helping to minimize pain and swelling.

- **Minimized Scarring:** By promoting healthy tissue regrowth, LED therapy can result in reduced scarring and better cosmetic outcomes for wounds.

- **Wound Types:** LED Light Therapy can be used for various wound types, including surgical incisions, burns, and injuries.

For specific wound healing cases, it's essential to follow the guidance of a healthcare professional or a wound care specialist. LED therapy can be a complementary treatment in many cases but should be used in conjunction with other wound care protocols for the best results.

CHAPTER 7

Combining LED Light Therapy with Other Skincare Treatments

7.1 Skincare Products

Combining LED Light Therapy with the right skincare products can enhance the overall effectiveness of your skincare routine. Here's how you can effectively incorporate skincare products with LED therapy:

- **Cleansing:** Start with a gentle, hydrating cleanser to remove makeup, dirt, and pollutants from your skin. Clean skin ensures that LED light penetrates effectively. Avoid harsh cleansers that may irritate your skin.

- **Exfoliation:** Depending on your skin type and concerns, consider using an exfoliant. Exfoliating before your LED session can help remove dead skin cells, allowing the light to reach deeper layers of the skin. However, be cautious with aggressive exfoliation, as LED therapy may increase skin sensitivity.

- **Serums and Topicals:** After your LED session, apply targeted skincare serums or topicals. LED therapy can enhance the absorption of these products, making them more effective. For example:

- **Vitamin C Serums:** These can help brighten the skin and improve collagen production.

- **Hyaluronic Acid Serums:** These provide hydration and can be particularly beneficial after LED therapy.

- **Retinoids:** If your dermatologist recommends retinoids for concerns like fine lines and wrinkles, use them as directed, typically in the evening, separate from your LED sessions.

- **Moisturizer:** Apply a suitable moisturizer to keep your skin hydrated. This step is especially important after LED therapy, as it can help lock in the benefits of the treatment.

- **Sunscreen:** Always apply sunscreen as the final step in your morning skincare routine. LED therapy can make your skin more sensitive to UV radiation, so protection is crucial.

- **Eye Cream:** If you're targeting specific eye area concerns, such as dark circles or puffiness, consider using an eye cream as part of your skincare routine.

- **Prescribed Medications:** If you have specific skin conditions that require prescribed medications, such as acne or rosacea, use them according to your dermatologist's instructions.

LED therapy can complement these treatments by enhancing their absorption.

Important Tips:

- **Consultation:** Consult with a dermatologist or skincare professional to select the right products for your skin type and concerns. They can help you create a personalized regimen that works well with LED therapy.

- **Timing:** For optimal results, apply skincare products after your LED session. The increased absorption during and immediately after LED therapy can enhance the effectiveness of your products.

- **Patch Testing:** If you're introducing new products to

your routine, perform a patch
test on a small area of your skin
to ensure there are no adverse
reactions.

- **Consistency:** Be consistent
  with your skincare routine and
  LED therapy. Consistency is
  key in achieving and
  maintaining results.

- **Avoid Harsh Products:** Avoid
  harsh or abrasive products that
  may irritate your skin when
  using LED therapy. Gentle and
  soothing products are generally
  recommended.

By thoughtfully combining LED
Light Therapy with the right skincare
products, you can enhance your
skincare routine, address specific
concerns, and maintain healthy,
radiant skin. Always follow the

recommendations of your healthcare professional or dermatologist for the most effective and safe approach to skincare and LED therapy.

7.2 Microneedling

Microneedling, also known as collagen induction therapy, involves using a device with fine needles to create controlled micro-injuries in the skin. This stimulates collagen and elastin production, leading to improved skin texture and reduced signs of aging. Combining microneedling with LED Light Therapy can be a powerful approach to rejuvenating the skin.

Why Combine Microneedling with LED Light Therapy:

1. **Enhanced Collagen Stimulation:** Both microneedling and LED therapy stimulate collagen production. Combining them can provide a synergistic effect, leading to more significant improvements in skin firmness and texture.

2. **Faster Healing:** LED therapy, particularly red and near-infrared light, can speed up the healing process following microneedling. It can reduce redness and inflammation, allowing you to recover more quickly.

3. **Reduced Side Effects:** The calming and anti-inflammatory properties of LED therapy can help reduce potential side

effects of microneedling, such as redness and swelling.

How to Combine Microneedling with LED Light Therapy:

1. **Microneedling Session:** Start with a microneedling session as recommended by your skincare professional. This typically involves the use of a microneedling device to create micro-injuries in the skin.

2. **LED Light Therapy:** After the microneedling session, apply LED Light Therapy using a red or near-infrared light source. This can be done immediately following microneedling or in the days that follow to assist with the healing process.

3. **Skincare Products:** Following your LED session, apply

calming and hydrating skincare products, as directed by your skincare professional.

4. **Sun Protection:** Always apply sunscreen after any skincare treatment. Both microneedling and LED therapy can make your skin more sensitive to UV radiation.

Important Tips:

- Always seek professional guidance when considering microneedling, as it requires specific training and expertise.

- Consult with your skincare professional to determine the most appropriate timing and schedule for combining microneedling and LED therapy.

- Be diligent about post-treatment care and follow the instructions provided by your skincare professional.

7.3 Chemical Peels

Chemical peels involve the application of a chemical solution to the skin to exfoliate the top layer, leading to skin rejuvenation. Combining chemical peels with LED Light Therapy can yield enhanced results in various skin concerns.

Why Combine Chemical Peels with LED Light Therapy:

1. **Improved Skin Rejuvenation:** LED therapy can enhance the effects of chemical peels by promoting collagen production and reducing inflammation,

leading to smoother, more radiant skin.

2. **Reduced Downtime:** LED therapy can help speed up the healing process after a chemical peel, minimizing redness and discomfort, and allowing you to resume your regular activities more quickly.

How to Combine Chemical Peels with LED Light Therapy:

1. **Chemical Peel Session:** Start with a chemical peel session as recommended by your skincare professional. The type and strength of the chemical peel will depend on your skin concerns.

2. **LED Light Therapy:** Following the chemical peel, apply LED Light Therapy using

appropriate wavelengths. The LED therapy can be applied either immediately after the peel or on subsequent days to assist with the healing process.

3. **Skincare Products:** After your LED session, apply soothing and hydrating skincare products to maintain the health of your newly exfoliated skin.

4. **Sun Protection:** Always use sunscreen to protect your skin after chemical peels and LED therapy, as your skin may be more sensitive to UV radiation.

Important Tips:

- Seek professional advice when considering chemical peels, as the type and strength of the peel should be determined by your skin type and concerns.

- Consult with your skincare professional to determine the most suitable timing and frequency for combining chemical peels and LED therapy.

- Be diligent about post-treatment care and adhere to the guidance provided by your skincare professional.

Thoughtfully combining treatments like microneedling or chemical peels with LED Light Therapy and following the recommendations of your skincare professional, you can achieve comprehensive skincare goals and maintain a radiant and youthful complexion.

CHAPTER 8

Maintenance and Aftercare

8.1 Post-Treatment Skin Care

Proper post-treatment care is essential to ensure your skin remains healthy and maintains the benefits of your LED Light Therapy and other skincare treatments.

- **After LED Therapy:** After an LED therapy session, apply a gentle and hydrating moisturizer to lock in the benefits. You may also apply any targeted serums or topicals recommended by your skincare professional.

- **After Microneedling or Chemical Peels:** Following microneedling or chemical peels, adhere to the specific aftercare instructions provided by your skincare professional. This may include the use of specialized post-treatment products and avoiding sun exposure and harsh skincare products.

- **Sun Protection:** Always apply sunscreen when going outside, as your skin may be more sensitive to UV radiation after LED therapy and certain skincare treatments. Sun protection is crucial for maintaining your results and preventing sun damage.

- **Hydration:** Keep your skin well-hydrated by using a suitable moisturizer. Hydrated skin is healthy skin.

- **Gentle Cleansing:** Continue to cleanse your skin with a gentle, non-alcoholic cleanser to remove dirt, sweat, and environmental pollutants. Avoid harsh cleansing products that may irritate your skin.

8.2 Tracking Progress

It's important to monitor your progress to determine the effectiveness of your skincare regimen, including LED Light Therapy and any additional treatments. Here's how you can track your progress:

- **Before and After Photos:** Take before and after photos in consistent lighting to visually assess changes in your skin's appearance. This can help you notice subtle improvements that may not be immediately apparent.

- **Journaling:** Keep a skincare journal to document changes in your skin, such as reduced acne breakouts, improved skin texture, or a reduction in hyperpigmentation.

- **Consult with a Professional:** Regularly consult with a dermatologist or skincare professional to evaluate your progress and make any necessary adjustments to your skincare routine.

- **Feedback from Others:**
  Friends and family may also
  notice changes in your skin.
  Their observations can be a
  valuable source of feedback.

8.3 Maintenance Routine

A maintenance routine is crucial to
preserve the results of your skincare
treatments and LED Light Therapy
over time. Here's how to establish an
effective maintenance routine:

- **Consistency:** Continue to be
  consistent with your LED Light
  Therapy sessions, skincare
  products, and any additional
  treatments.

- **Follow Professional Advice:**
  Consult with a skincare
  professional for guidance on

adjusting your routine as needed to address changing skincare concerns or goals.

- **Update Your Products:** As your skin's needs change, update your skincare products to ensure they are still suitable for your skin type and concerns.

- **Regular Skin Checks:** Perform regular skin self-checks and monitor any changes in your skin. If you notice any unusual moles, spots, or skin conditions, consult with a dermatologist.

- **Lifestyle Habits:** Maintain a healthy lifestyle with good hydration, a balanced diet, regular exercise, and adequate sleep to support overall skin health.

- **Stress Management:** Manage stress, as it can impact your skin's condition. Practices like meditation and relaxation techniques can be beneficial.

- **Professional Treatments:** Continue to schedule periodic professional treatments, such as microneedling or chemical peels, to maintain your skin's health and address specific concerns.

Implementing a thorough aftercare routine, consistently tracking your progress, and establishing a maintenance regimen, you can enjoy long-lasting benefits from your LED Light Therapy and other skincare treatments while maintaining healthy, radiant skin.